Pathemata

ALSO BY MAGGIE NELSON

Like Love

On Freedom: Four Songs of Care and Constraint

The Argonauts

The Art of Cruelty: A Reckoning

Bluets

The Red Parts: Autobiography of a Trial

Women, the New York School, and Other True Abstractions

Something Bright, Then Holes

Jane: A Murder

The Latest Winter

Shiner

Pathemata

Or,
The Story of My Mouth

MAGGIE NELSON

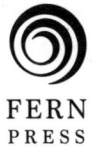

FERN
PRESS

1 3 5 7 9 10 8 6 4 2

Fern Press, an imprint of Vintage,
is part of the Penguin Random House group of companies

Vintage, Penguin Random House UK, One Embassy Gardens,
8 Viaduct Gardens, London SW11 7BW

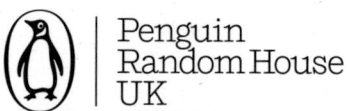

penguin.co.uk/vintage
global.penguinrandomhouse.com

First published by Fern Press in 2025
Copyright © Maggie Nelson 2025

Maggie Nelson has asserted her right to be identified as the author of this
Work in accordance with the Copyright, Designs and Patents Act 1988

Penguin Random House values and supports copyright. Copyright fuels creativity, encourages diverse voices, promotes freedom of expression and supports a vibrant culture. Thank you for purchasing an authorised edition of this book and for respecting intellectual property laws by not reproducing, scanning or distributing any part of it by any means without permission. You are supporting authors and enabling Penguin Random House to continue to publish books for everyone. No part of this book may be used or reproduced in any manner for the purpose of training artificial intelligence technologies or systems. In accordance with Article 4(3) of the DSM Directive 2019/790, Penguin Random House expressly reserves this work from the text and data mining exception.

Typeset in 11.25/16.56 pt Fournier MT Pro by Jouve (UK), Milton Keynes
Printed and bound in Great Britain by Clays Ltd, Elcograf S.p.A.

The authorised representative in the EEA is Penguin Random House Ireland,
Morrison Chambers, 32 Nassau Street, Dublin D02 YH68

A CIP catalogue record for this book is available from the British Library

HB ISBN 9781911717454

Penguin Random House is committed to a sustainable future
for our business, our readers and our planet. This book is made
from Forest Stewardship Council® certified paper.

I get up first to be alone, and also because my jaw hurts too much to stay in bed.
Each morning it is as if my mouth has survived a war – it has protested, it has hidden, it has suffered.
It has floated, its minuscule points of contact have hit and repelled, pain has shocked then pooled up around the joint.
Rather than each other, my teeth find cheek, which they masticate, leaving in their wake two mountainous ridges.
I shove the sheet into my mouth to know that I am still here, still rooted to the crust.

When H is home, which is about half of the time these days,
I apologise to him for the white splotches on the comforter's rim.
He says it's okay, they just make him sad.
As I tiptoe to the kitchen, I 'bite check', which I've been instructed not to do, but I do it anyway, to make sure my top and bottom teeth are still in the same mouth, lost cousins of the same star.

He has pulled the car over on a rural highway to help a turtle cross the road.

We are on a blind incline, so there is a significant risk of them both getting hit by an oncoming car.

He treats the turtle with tenderness and urgency, more tenderness and urgency than he has ever shown toward me.

I wait in the passenger seat, watching the heat steam off the asphalt.

I don't care if the turtle lives, but I pretend that I do.

I am trying to be loved.

There is a window of time, right after waking, when the mind is allegedly freshest for creating.

An article in the paper calls it 'the morning rush'.

For about two years I kill it, by reading the news on Twitter.

First I get to know the personalities and dogs and knitting habits of ex-prosecutors.

I marvel at their ease with moral language – this, after years spent putting people in cages.

Then I spend time with various epidemiologists, getting to know their senses of humour, their compulsions ('just staying for Omicron!'), their punctuation styles, their 'risk tolerance', their wounded response to the aggression of others.

I particularly enjoy Monica Gandhi's embattled optimism, her passive-aggressive 'thanks', her nearly erotic appreciation of the vaccines.

Orofacial pain clinic number one can't help.
Orofacial pain clinic number two can't help.
As I set off into the uninsured wilds, I start a file on my desktop, wherein I catalogue the conditions of the pain's onset, the doctors I've seen, the results of their imaging, the medications and physical therapies I've tried, the activities that seem to make it better and worse, and so on.
I bring this document to each new appointment, hoping it might offer a useful summary of a confusing physical situation, as well as confirm my status as an organised patient eager to participate in her treatment.

We are driving along East Blithedale in the dark in a van, Grandpa at the wheel.
He is silhouetted, and we know we are in trouble.
We are en route to the scene of the crime, but what crime?

When we get there it's the girls' room in *The Brady Bunch*.
An ex-student is walking around with her cancerous cleft lip, talking
about trauma, calling it the 'fuckfestivity'.
There the mother among us has a psychedelic moment in which
her skull turns into radiant phosphenes with horrifying cavernous
teeth – it signifies her guilt for having let her husband,
my grandfather, torture and kill his daughter, and for her having
kept his secret all these years.

It doesn't take me long to realise that no one wants to read this
pathemata.
People flick through it, then tuck it into the rear of my file,
as if its principal message were that I am a logorrhoeic in need
of management.

My file begins with a flu I'd had at my grandfather's funeral,
an unusual flu that brought a month-long fever, and left as its
residue a certain difficulty in swallowing.
From there the symptoms literally branch out: electric threads along
my lower gum, a snake of pain looping from jaw to eye, a constant,
kinetic ache in the joint, the recurring feeling that I had received a
blow to the face while sleeping.

Not wanting to miss any details that might prove key, I allow
the tapestry to widen, weaving in my early history with speech
therapy, lifelong struggles with tonsillitis, adolescent adventures
in orthodonture, previous barium swallows and bouts of TMJ, the
weaning of my baby, perimenopause, domestic stressors, the literal
and symbolic role of the mouth in the life of a writer.

When he comes for me, it isn't him any more – it's a Victorian kewpie
doll with an updo wearing a mustard-coloured dress.
Her pubic hair is visible through the dress, a stringy mound.
I grab my treasure chest of Dad's silver dollars to pummel her with,
but when I reach up, I can only reach the mound.

I tell H about the horrible reveal that my grandfather was his
daughter's murderer.
He assures me that bad dreams are mental detritus signifying
nothing, forget about it, go back to sleep.
This dismissal, which I know he intends as a comfort, enrages me.
It enrages me so much that I get up and write down my dream.

As a kid I talked so much and at such high velocity that I had to go to speech therapy so that people could better understand me.
I could, of course, understand myself perfectly – as could my sister – so part of me wondered whether there was something else they wanted to fix, which they were euphemistically calling 'my mouth'.
'Does her mouth come with an off switch?' a family friend once joked after taking care of me for the weekend – the kind of flip joke between adults that ends up sticking with you for the rest of your life (and the kind that I have surely made at least one of by now, even if I didn't intend to).

My fast speech was apparently complicated by a 'tongue thrust', a situation that an auburn-moustached orthodontist – since deceased – tried to fix by gluing a metal spike to the back of my front teeth.
The goal, I gathered, was to intimidate my tongue into finding a different place to create sibilance (*but where?*).
Each time I heard the adults say 'thrust' it sounded fat and lewd, like Jabba the Hutt.

I'm trying to get to a dentist appointment at which they are finally going to fix my mouth.
H is driving me, as a courtesy. But he hasn't looked up the directions.

By the time we get across town he's driving up weird hills instead of staying straight on Santa Monica Boulevard.
I'm so frustrated, it's 4.20 for a 4 p.m. appointment, now getting close to 5, we're going to miss it.
We pull over at a train station, we're now in France, there is a little gift shop with a lot of doilies and stuff shrink-wrapped in plastic, plus brioche.
I try to buy a ticket from a machine but my American twenty keeps getting rejected.
I'm angry now, and trying to download an app I need to contact the office.
It's called BREATHE DENTISTRY, and I can't get it to load.

The metal spike delivered its message – my tongue was wrong – its *instincts* were wrong.
As was its size.
I imagined shaving it down into something thinner and more elegant, as one might whittle a walking stick from a log.
But a tongue can't be whittled.
A tongue is bloody and strong.

We're in some kind of public setting, maybe a classroom, and H says, I've decided that this person is really interesting to me, and I'm not going to hold back any more, I'm going to go on a date.
Someone in the room says, You're not even thirty days sober, don't you think you should wait?
I say, Sober? What about the fact that you're married?
I see a text this person has sent him – it's very touchy-feely, jargon-filled – I think it's beneath him.
Yet it's so different from me, I can see its allure.
H says something about her ability to brainstorm, and I think to myself, I will never 'brainstorm', I will keep my ideas private until the last minute, I will never be what you desire.

Some musical guests from out of town are performing at our middle-school assembly; their music moves me.
It moves me so much that I have a flash that, if I stand up and start dancing, it might spark a *Fame*-like moment, as when the whole crowd bursts into 'Hot Lunch', or, better yet, 'I Sing the Body Electric'.
So up I sprout from the gymnasium floor, upon which everyone else is sitting, cross-legged.
I try to act cool by not quitting even after I realise I will be dancing alone, but after about five seconds – count them, this is an eternity of solo dancing in front of a junior high – I sit back down.

Later that day, my sister, who is in eighth grade, will tell me it was the most humiliating moment of her life.
How do you think it felt, all these faces turning to me, asking, 'Isn't that your *sister?'*
She walks home from the bus stop a block ahead of me, in punishment.

Quarantining at a house in the woods.
There are children running around and all the adults are languidly complaining about their marriages.
I'm wearing a robe that won't close in the front.
Someone keeps talking about Guided by Voices, who in this dream is a girlband.
I don't know who they mean.
One of the kids needs to nap. Liam or something.
I think how glad I am that I don't have to do it, put him down.

The same year I danced at the assembly, one of my sister's friends did a lip sync to 'Like a Virgin' in the drama room.
She wore a wedding dress, just like Madonna.
The part I liked most was when she started humping the floor.

When she started doing that, the authority figure in the room called the performance off.
Years later, I saw Britney Spears perform '. . . Baby One More Time' at an awards show, and I saw that she, too, had the humping spirit.
I liked it.
It's unhinged, grungy, like mould growing under the lid of a marinara jar.
I also worried for Britney, because I knew that that much energy is hard to manage.
I knew because I felt it too.
Mostly, I felt it in my mouth.

In speech therapy we played a board game in which to advance you had to say a tongue twister slowly and clearly.
The imperative to *slow down*, combined with my tongue's whimpering confusion each time it encountered the metal prick, produced in me a fear and fantasy that one day my tongue would simply rip free of its vassalage, like the Black Stallion cut loose to eat seaweed and run on the beach with traumatised, freckled Alec. Unspeared, it would produce such extraordinary speech that it wouldn't matter any more if the multitude could understand me – I would echolocate, and in time a tribe of like-tongued people – the humpers, the thrusters – would advance over the summit, leather-clad, to recover me.

Later, in a sauna, which is also a video-viewing room at a museum –
I'm still wearing the robe.
A guy pushes open the cedar door and starts commenting on
the asymmetry of a group of stuffed animals arranged on a dark
platform in the corner.
I ignore him.
Then I look over and realise he is naked, his huge cock lying against
his stomach.
I can't tell if I'm sixteen like I feel, or fifty.
My toes hang out at the end of my robe, monstrous.

I go see a Lyme doctor I find on the internet, a renowned one who
apparently treated Amy Tan.
He is in San Francisco and I fly there to see him.
It feels reckless but the pain keeps demanding an answer.
The waiting room is full of teenagers and old folks and everyone in
between; the mood is rigorous and sombre.
There are photos of ticks and newspaper articles about Lyme disease
all over the walls.
It reminds me of Saratoga Springs, a place I once went thinking it
would be a bourgeois hippie spa with aromatherapy candles and
womb-like treatment rooms, but instead felt like an insane asylum
where you'd go to get electric shock – teal and white cinderblock
walls, porcelain-enamelled tubs, brisk employees.

I don't feel at all sure that my pain is tick-related, but I did spend seven consecutive summers in tick country and half the people I know from there are on canes or IVs, and everyone I talk to about my pain keeps asking if I have investigated the Lyme angle, so I figure I should give it a shot.

In my teens and early twenties I never wanted to put my own finger inside me because I knew I would think something was wrong.
Then I didn't have that feeling for a long time.
I have it again now.
I felt some weird bony muscle in there a few years ago that felt like a tree branch knocked awry and I freaked out.
I've long been haunted by that scene in a Harmony Korine movie when two teens are making out and he's feeling her up and then he's like, What's this lump?
I think it might even cut to her funeral.
Which is weird because I'm not really sure teenage girls get breast cancer.

At the first appointment the Lyme doctor does a lot of bloodwork.
At the second, just as I suspected, he is convinced that I have Lyme, even though the bloodwork is inconclusive.
He says because the bloodwork has returned a positive for another tick infection, albeit not an active one, it's really a slam dunk that I also have Lyme and that the disease is attacking the nerves in my face and mouth.
I express reservations about taking antibiotics or other drugs without a firmer diagnosis and he says with irritation, Do you want to go on living with the pain, or do you want to treat it and have it go away?
I'm shivering in a white paper gown when he hands me the prescription for doxy.

Exhausted by reality TV and appalled by the replacements for Alex Trebek, my son and I embark on *The Brady Bunch* from Season One.
I find many things about the experience strange, one of which being how I used to identify with Jan, and now I identify primarily with Alice.
I also see how compelling it is that the parents don't seem to have any other interests save their children, and that they always work together.
They are 'on the same page', their authority gentle but absolute.

Also, to make it a comedy, no one communicates clearly, and that is fine – necessary, even.
Each episode depends upon a secret or lie or omission, so that, in the end, something can be found out.

The doxy stains my teeth but that's about it. My jaw still hurts.
When he suggests we move to Seroquel, I know I won't return.
I end up feeling ashamed of the whole adventure, though I do feel glad that now, when well-meaning people say, *Bear with me here, but have you ever thought about Lyme?*, I can tell them that I have been treated for Lyme, and it didn't make the pain go away.
But now my front teeth are streaked with brown stripes, so I have to find someone willing to grind the stains off.

In last night's episode, none of the Brady kids tells the parents that, earlier in the day, they broke a vase and glued it back together, so at dinner the kids watch the vase warily until water starts sprouting through the cracks – that's the tension, the comedy, the reveal.
It was weird because, earlier that day, I had been thinking about *The Golden Bowl* – in particular, about how I had long remembered the novel as a parable about good enough containers, like good enough

mothering, or good enough works of art, but, upon re-examination, I see that James is talking about marriage.

A marriage with a crack.

A surly teen has been dragged to a family Christmas; from the moment he exits the Subaru Outback, he stays glued to his phone. Everyone begs him to put it down and join in the rituals of family life – at one point his grandpa even throws a sock at his face, to disrupt him.

The teen refuses, can barely look away long enough to hang a single ornament.

At the end of the commercial, he assembles his family in the living room, and screens for them the movie he's been secretly filming for the past several days.

The movie features his relatives trading affection, the children making snow angels, and the reverse shot of the sock hurling at his lens.

It makes everyone laugh and cry.

The family embraces the teen and recognises, at long last, his indispensable contribution to the fold.

Nearly all the artists I know, especially the householders, harbour some version of this fantasy.

In the shower I lather my boobs with soap, and remind myself that I don't have to examine them for lumps every day just because the soap makes them slick.

I think about how grateful I am for all they've given me – exquisite sensation, almost enough to come by, milk given freely and extracted roughly, a certain shape in clothes.

But as more and more friends have theirs removed, be it by choice or to stay alive, I sometimes feel a longing to join them.

Those who would call this a mutilation would seem to have an investment in stasis and a fear of regret that I do not share.

My favourite moment from any interview ever:

What has been your biggest disappointment?

I don't think it's an interesting question, forgive me (John Cage).

C is going to heaven – a thought that gripped me when I was nineteen, when C was my feminist theory teacher.

This conviction was odd, in that I am not religious, do not believe in an afterlife, and have never bought into the idea that the souls of queers or feminists or Marxist scholars – all of which C was – are a priori endangered, not even a little bit.

But there was something about C – her essential goodness, the laser of her presence, her plain-spoken righteousness (no doubt derived from her upbringing – unknown to me at the time – as an

Anabaptist) – that stood in such contrast to the homophobic bigots all around us, that 'heaven' kept popping into my mind in her presence, a marble rolled in from someone else's game.
To celebrate my senior thesis – a Foucauldian analysis of *aveu* in Sexton and Plath – she took me to a normcore restaurant on the river, wherein she proposed a toast 'to rigour'.

Looking for a friend who no longer answers my texts at a grimy amusement park.
I finally find her, she has sores on her face and is clearly a junkie.
I'm like, so this is why she hasn't wanted to talk to me.
She has short new wave hair, says it's all okay, she has a therapist now.

I feel a lot of pain when I think about the suicide of Nicholas Hughes, Sylvia Plath's son.
At the time of his death he was forty-seven, an expert in salmon biology living in Fairbanks, Alaska.
I didn't know how important it was to me that Plath's children were still alive until I heard the news of Nicholas's death, which crushed me.

When he was an infant, Plath wrote to him: 'The blood blooms
clean // In you, ruby. / The pain / You wake to is not yours.'
I've been reading these words, composed by Plath in her dark
winter, for nearly four decades now.
They mean more to me now – they *hurt* more now – than ever
before.
When did her pain become his?
Or is it unfair not to treat his pain as his own?

In the good script I am supermom going to vaccinate my child after
all this time to protect him and make everything okay.
In the bad script the clinic at the Children's Hospital tells me they
have closed for the day, but I can come back in the morning to get
his second shot.
I have driven over an hour across town in traffic for an appointment
with *this* time written on the confirmation email, and feel sure
that we need to get the shot *today*, as so instructed, so instead of
just letting it go and coming back in the morning, I consult the
government website on my phone, which tells me to go to a clinic in
Glendale.
The clinic in Glendale turns out to be a suburban hellhole – dank
carpet no windows crying children febrile-seeming assholes reading
their phones with their masks hanging below their chins.

The admin lady ensconced in a plexiglas box won't tell me if they have the paediatric vaccine, she just keeps telling me to wait.
We wait, we wait.
I grow more and more exasperated, flushed with the determination to give my son this final protection, and fear that my determination is precisely what will infect him.
After an hour, the lady in the box confesses that they're waiting to see if any other kids show up, in which case they'll dethaw some kids' vaccine.
I demand my paperwork back and leave in a huff, abusing the elevator buttons on our way down.

The government website now says, Go to a Pasadena Vons.
At the Pasadena Vons they say Try the Sierra Madre Vons.
At the Sierra Madre Vons they say Yes, but only on Fridays.
I make one last stop at the CVS near our house 'just to see' and by now my son is begging me to stop.
Just stop, Mom.

I go see a dentist in the valley recommended to me by both my acupuncturist and chiropractor, two strong women I respect – one Korean, the other Swiss – with offices on opposite sides of town.

That they don't know each other but have given me the same name feels like a sign.

The waiting room of his office is slick beyond belief, with video testimonials of people whose jaw pain he has supposedly cured playing on large monitors.

The people in the videos say everything I want to be able to say: *I had almost given up, the treatment was a godsend, I have my life back, I ate a hamburger for the first time in years, I can finally get a good night's sleep.*

I wonder, if he cures my pain, if I would assent to starring in one of these videos, the way I once let the City University of New York make a poster of me testifying to the institution's greatness.

The poster hung in an elevator in the main lobby at 365 Fifth Avenue – an elevator I then avoided for the next two years, letting people board without me while I waited for one that didn't feature my face, even though I knew no one was really looking at the posters or at me and even if they were, who cares.

We get home without the second shot and in penance I let my son eat some donuts left over from my class.

He tells me how awful it is when I get angry and I tell him he's right.

I have never felt as angry as I've felt over the past two years.

I tell him that even though it looks like I'm a hot mess driving all over town begging for one little orange-topped vial of Pfizer, I'm really more like the mom in the animated movie we just watched who says *I have made the metal ones pay for their crimes* while wiping robot blood from her face.

He doesn't respond, as he is busy roving Hyrule, killing Bokoblins, harvesting opals.

At least nothing bad happens in *Zelda*, he says.

You die over and over again in *Zelda*, I say back.

The dentist in the valley turns out to be a squat Italian brunet in his thirties whom I immediately distrust.

After his female assistants put a visor on me and run a red laser over my jaw for fifteen minutes, he makes a theatrical entrance, announcing, Today we're not only going to tell you why you've been in so much pain, we're going to show you.

We do a bunch of imaging and he starts to point things out, but he's rushing and I don't see what he sees.

It sounds like he's giving the same speech he's given many times before, and I marvel at my inability to know if the whole thing is a hoax, how the intensity of my desire to get out of pain vies with my intelligence, which, on a good day, I consider formidable.

He concludes by saying, If you pay the 5K up front, we'll take
moulds for your appliances right now, and you'll get out of pain that
much faster.
He says the appliances take six weeks to come back from the lab, so
it's best to start right away.
Even though it's been years, the sound of six more weeks makes
tears involuntarily sprout from my eyes, so I say okay.

At the minimart, examining packages of Certs and bottles of
AriZona iced tea.
An artist-hustler approaches and flashes open his jacket, revealing a
giant, log-sized syringe strapped to the interior flap.
He acts as if it's some great humanitarian offering, but I decline,
saying the research isn't in yet.

The decision to work with the dentist in the valley proves fateful.
I visit him for months, wear his appliances.
He places little slips of paper between my top and bottom teeth
to track their contact while explaining that he rejects pharmaceutical
contracts because he's 'not interested in blowjobs from

supermodels', and that, if he needs to make extra money, he serves as an expert witness in court cases having to do with people's mouths.

Later I write him an email telling him that his remarks about the blowjobs made me uncomfortable.

He writes back and says that he's mortified, that he felt 'just a bit too comfortable' with me.

He signs his email 'with love and gratitude'.

I consider writing him again to say that his sign-off also feels inappropriate, but I'm tired.

I feel the way I often feel with sexists, like, I could mop the floor with them, but also, I'm finding some rapport.

And perhaps out of necessity, as I've paid up front for relief he may or may not have to offer.

I wake up and write down the sentence, *I dreamt I was in a room with pink walls and an* Equus *poster*.

The sentence thrills me – it's as if a rough paw has swiped through my brain and emerged with this dab of jelly.

Equus was a big play when I was little.

I wasn't allowed to see it, but I knew it had to do with a naked teenage boy stabbing his eyes out, like Oedipus, in a stable.

At some point I learned that the boy spikes out the eyes of six horses

and not his own, but it was too late – now I had two unthinkable scenarios upon which to cogitate.
The book sat on a low shelf of my parents' paperbacks, next to *Jaws* and *The World According to Garp*.
The combination titillated and bewildered me, as I knew it mixed together a woman marching to her dismemberment after night-time lovemaking on the beach, her boobs glowing like two globes of bait; a group of women who cut out their tongues in solidarity with a little girl whose rapist had performed the same mutilation on her; and a forbidden mélange of nudity, ice picks, horses and therapy.

Now that I've written all this down, *I dreamt I was in a room with pink walls and an* Equus *poster* doesn't sound so random.
It sounds like an invagination – a chamber to hold the pastiche of lacerations.

My teeth keep moving.
Eventually they lose all contact, save two tiny points at the back.
When I stand in mountain pose, I no longer feel a connection to the mothership.
I experiment with what I can hold between my teeth: a pencil is big enough; a thinning cough drop is not.
Eating salad becomes a joke.

I can chew meat until the edges are softened but I can no longer break it down.

I wonder if there are bad health effects from not chewing your food, besides choking.

Mr Goodbody – well-intentioned, disturbing creature of 1970s TV, who looked like Richard Simmons (*was* he Richard Simmons?) – thought so.

Poor Mr Goodbody, in his pantyhose bodysuit with all the organs painted atop, his numbles on forever display.

Though why the pity?

Mr Goodbody was spry and cheerful, a pedagogue.

If anything, he shamed others, or at least warned them – as when he made a slit under a rib and fished out a two-inch piece of unchewed meat with a wire.

The sternness with which he displayed the soggy grey jerky to the children made clear that he considered it an abomination, a horror.

I will think of this jerky when a friend tells me that she recently took a medication that had the unexpected side effect of depleting her gastric acid – she knew something was awry because her waste started coming out looking like complete meals, each morsel recognisable for what it had been when it went in.

It was like you could put it on a plate and serve it, she said.

If I wake up before 5 a.m., I stuff the sheet between my teeth and try to go back to sleep, using all my mantras: *Imagine yourself healthy, happy and free. You are home, you are loved, you are safe.*
One morning, in a tiny miracle, I succeed in sleeping in for two more hours, during which time I dream I wrote a book with the word *Pensées* on the cover in cursive pastels.
I wake up delighted – I finally wrote something funny.

The dentist in the valley and I go back and forth over injecting my jaw with Botox.
I hold out, realising that the only thing that frightens me more than pain and its viciousness is numbness, paralysis.

I go see someone about my mouth at a home office in Pasadena: quiet residential street with no sidewalks, green lawns, rich-seeming.
The woman is a retired myofascial therapist, or something like that – I've lost track of who recommended that I see her.
She's a petite white lady in her sixties, short grey hair, muscly.
We talk a bit, after which she tells me she's been making small talk in order to observe my mouth.
She says that if she walked into a party and saw me from across

the room she would know immediately that I have an open bite, a tongue thrust, a history of speech problems, and could likely use a frenectomy.

I find this unnerving, as I speak in public all the time – sometimes on jumbo screens, and now on Zoom, which stipulates more facial exposure than anyone, save those who have signed up for a career in cinema or TV, deserves.

I am a visiting writer somewhere and the more esteemed visiting writer – who arrives with the reputation of a playboy – is trying to make time for me.

He has a mouth condition wherein a bluish, bad-smelling ink periodically floods the flower of his tongue.

It's some kind of blood disease, people say.

I go down on my knees to give him a blowjob, but he isn't hard, his pants are just grey, creased softness in the crotch.

I don't take it personally, I feel a kind of pity.

He holds a long seagull feather in front of his mouth to indicate when the affliction is in – the feather's vane turns orange when the smelly ink comes around.

The Pasadena lady and I talk frenulum surgery.
She says it will be tremendously liberating, but that I will need help learning to talk afterwards.
She says I will need to take time off from public speaking, during which she would train me to gain control over my tongue, which would be, post-surgery, akin to the unmanned spurting hose I'd always feared and imagined.

My first troll in the chat.
She wishes I would stop talking so much and let my co-panellist talk more.
I'm trying to stay focused but she's growing incensed, starting to use all caps.
WHY WON'T ANYONE RESPOND TO ME???!!
The moderator writes, *We will definitely respond to you, but I can't quite find the question here. Can you rephrase?*
I'm astonished at the moderator's politeness.
Someone else writes, *She's not asking a question, she's making a comment. Please respond.*
A shadow event has opened up alongside the main event, and threatens to steal the show.

I wonder what I would learn about other people's mouths if I applied to them the same scrutiny.

I try it, and notice right off the bat that a lot of people have a problem opposite of mine – their teeth seem to touch too much, like maybe their top and bottom front teeth catch or grind.

This seems like a potentially worse problem, but I'm not sure if it causes them pain.

I marvel at the fact that some people with bites obviously more fucked up than mine have no pain, just like two people could have identical back MRIs but one can't get out of bed and the other does CrossFit.

I think about C's mouth – how it was ravaged in the accident, how her jaw was reconstructed, and how, when I first saw her after, she had metal bars across the roof of her mouth, to keep everything in place.

In the seventeen years that followed, I never heard her talk about mouth pain, maybe because she didn't have any, or maybe because she had more pain everywhere else.

Back at home, I watch YouTube videos of people post-frenectomy. They seem spiritually transported by how free they feel once their tongues have been unclipped.

Decades of neck pain evaporate overnight; the liberated weep with relief.
Many of the doctors in the videos remind viewers that, while the surgery may seem niche, in other countries, babies regularly have their frenulums snipped at birth, to facilitate nursing.
Doing it as an adult, they say, just frees and sets something right that could have been freed and set right long ago.

Not long after I begin my experiment of looking at other people's mouths, I quit it.
It feels intrusive and mean, and also like bad karma, if I don't want anyone looking at mine.

The Pasadena therapist recommends that I get started on my path to frenectomy by seeing a dentist she works with, whose name she scrawls on the back of her card.
He ends up being a strange man in his seventies who works as a team with his wife in matching white coats – he talks and does the exam while she sits on a high stool at a computer, poking information into the machine.
I say strange because he is preppy in a loafers/pink skin/combed

white hair kind of way, but his evangelism about the virtues of frenectomy feels unusual, cultish.

After evaluating my mouth, he surprises me by telling me he does not think I'm a strong candidate for the surgery.

Says I'm only moderately tongue-tied, and that he doesn't think it will relieve my pain.

I am unused to people not pushing the procedures they are selling.

Instead, he suggests that I start taping my mouth shut when I sleep.

He tells me that he and his wife have been taping their mouths shut for years, and he can't emphasise enough how much it has improved their sleep, and their life more generally.

She smiles and bobs her head in agreement, as if this night-time taping has been the key to their marriage's success.

I imagine them kissing in their white coats, mouths taped shut, like Magritte's enshrouded lovers.

Months after my visit to the Pasadena therapist, I get a voicemail from a young woman who says that she is the therapist's daughter, and that she's very sorry for the delay, but that she's just now getting around to calling everyone in her mother's call history.

Her tone indicates that her mother is dead, though she doesn't say so directly.

When H is home, I hear him haunting the premises all night.
Each activity – popcorn popping, the clatter of violence on Netflix, the crack of an aluminum can – floats into my bedroom – our bedroom – like a fresh abandonment.
As the pandemic drags on, he goes to bed later and later and I get up earlier and earlier, until we approach the singularity.
At dawn I pick up cigarette butts and crushed cans from the yard, wipe pizza crumbs off the counter, as if cleaning up after a rager to which I wasn't invited.

Try not to think of it as, *Your tongue is too big for your mouth*, but rather, *Your palate is too narrow for your tongue*, the mouth-taping dentist had said.
I was unsure how this was supposed to make me feel better, but I did enjoy the novel pleasure of embracing my tongue for a few days, and shifting the blame onto my palate instead.
(*What is a palate, anyway?*)
It reminded me of when doctors would express concern about the size of my baby *in utero*, and the woman we'd hired to assist my birth would say, *Don't worry – women don't tend to make babies they can't get out.*
This was reassuring, and helped me get through labour with what turned out to be a truly huge baby.

It was also probably inaccurate — babies clog up the works, rip women apart, all the time.

H and I are trying to kill each other with butter knives.
We are in bed, the light is black and gold.
The question is, Will one of us really try to put a butter knife through the other's heart?
Our knives duel weakly over his bare chest.

In order not to lose the money I spent buying a six-month gym membership, I have to tell the owner what kind of injury has kept me from coming to class.
I tell her a little, trying to act nonchalant, and not like someone who keeps a 10,000-word pain history on her desktop.
She says she has just the person for me, someone who worked miracles on her after she was injured in a car crash.
She says she knows it will seem woo-woo, but really, I should trust her — this is the kind of person who can help when no one else has been able to.
I go see this body worker, and lie in her pleasant, cream-coloured studio while she does unthinkably subtle touching around my jaw, neck and pelvis.

It's pleasant enough, but nothing shifts.

After about six visits, she tells me that she doesn't think it's ethical to keep taking my money if it's not working (a fertility nurse once told me the same thing).

At this point in the treatment, she says, her preference would be to take a Polaroid of me to send to her guru in Minneapolis, who, she attests, has the astonishing power to diagnose what's wrong with someone just from looking at their picture.

Recently he could tell that someone had advanced cancer before she even knew anything was wrong, she says.

This sounds perfectly ghastly to me, the exact opposite of the kind of care I'd been seeking.

Yet somehow I feel I have to assent to this plan to get out of her studio.

I pose for the mugshot, my cheeks burning with weakness.

He's a genius, you'll see, she says, stripping my likeness out of the antiquated machine. *It'll just take a couple of weeks.*

Sometimes I wonder what I would have thought about all these years, if I hadn't spent so much time thinking about the pain.

Then I remember that I've thought about a lot of other things as well.

Also, I'm not sure the goal of life is to think about as many things as possible.

I have been splashed all over with mud and I'm lowering myself into a silty shallow river to try to get clean, a fool's errand.
It has to do with H, like I'm preparing to mount him, so we can move together up the river like an alligator carrying her baby on her studs.
We are deep in the woods.

A couple of weeks go by, then a couple of months.
I confess to H what transpired, tell him I'm scared the guru divined something so horrible from my Polaroid that the body worker felt unable to get back in touch with me.
He is incredulous that I have let myself go down this path, as am I.
The whole thing brings to mind a relationship I had in the mid-nineties with a guy who, when he broke up with me, confessed he'd been shooting up and sleeping on and off with his room-mate, who worked as an escort.
In the weeks and months that followed, I became consumed by the thought that only he knew whether he'd transmitted HIV to me – that only he had this critical knowledge about my well-being that I needed, but couldn't get without talking to him again, which I knew would be profoundly unwise.
I also knew that, even if he had the information to give, it wouldn't make the infection or the chance of infection go away; the problem would still be mine.

I'm waiting in line for an aesthetician with a blonde bob to paint my face with slip.
The paintbrush is fat, the slip pale yellow.
Her beauty and nonchalance contrast terribly with what she's up to – the slip is preparation for burning my face off; the next stop is a kiln.
When my turn comes I beg her not to do it – I am unsure if, if I die here, I will die everywhere.
But she's unreachable, a true *Margarete*.

It takes six months and a negative test from the free clinic on Essex for me to feel that I had gotten away from him for good, that I belonged to myself again, that he had nothing on me.

I never hear back from the body worker, but about a year later, I find myself behind her in the checkout line at Sprouts.
She says a furtive hello, like she is abashed, or can't place me.
For an instant I think – she's going to tell me now, right here in the checkout line, what her guru saw.
But then I realise that the thing I had feared most – that she was going to inform me of my imminent death – had not come to pass.
All this time, and I was still alive.

A couple is renewing their vows in the presence of all those who have ever threatened them; chairs for the ceremony have been arranged in concentric circles under a tin roof, ramshackle.
On my turn, I'm summoned to the innermost circle, so that everyone can behold 'the adulteress'.
I'm wearing a sundress with spaghetti straps, no mask.
Through tears of joy, the wife tells the crowd, 'When we're home together now, I finally feel safe.'
People throw roses after the couple as they leave in a Rolls-Royce – it's part wedding, part funeral, stunning in its meanness.
I mill around at the after-party, arguing that, while the couple may seem like today's winners, ours is the more literary position.

When the virus hits, I don't have a general practitioner; mine retired in January 2020 (impeccable timing, I can't help but think).
Sensing that it's not a great time to be without one, I pick a GP out of my university network and set up an online 'meet-and-greet'.
At the end of an awkward, blurry session which includes the GP telling me how she once saved her father-in-law's life by doing CPR on him after he'd had a heart attack in his sleep – a story she tells in response to my disclosure that my father died of a heart attack in his – she asks me if, were I to fall ill, there is anything I would like to communicate to those I'd left behind, as sometimes doctors keep such things on file.

I am taken aback – is she asking for my last words?
No, no, she says, it's not like that, it's just about whether there is anything I'd like her to have on file.
I tell her I'll think about it, then hang up feeling a hundred times more distressed than I'd felt before the call.

One day *The Brady Bunch* disappears from Hulu, without a trace.
That happens sometimes, H shrugs.
I'm crestfallen that my son and I won't get to the end of the story, as if there were one.

I tell my therapist about the meet-and-greet, and ask her if she thinks I should write down some words for my son in case I die suddenly of Covid.
No, she says, I do *not* think that is a good idea for you.
I'm surprised by her adamance, though she sometimes gets this way when I tell her about things other licensed health professionals have said.
However, she says, she had been thinking of a different exercise for me – how would I feel about writing myself a letter, from my dead father, in his voice as well as I can remember it?

Just to see what he might have to say to me now?
I am not in the habit of writing in response to therapeutic prompts, and feel quite certain that my imitation of my father's voice would be a humiliation to me as a writer.
But, diligent student that I am, I attempt it later that afternoon.

I am wearing a black crop top and perusing the goods at an outdoor flea market when I feel a hand snake around my bare waist and another lock over my mouth.
Right away I know I am being abducted.
Promptly, I split from my body – I look down and see my feet being lifted out of someone else's beat-up Chelsea boots.
I know that the abductors are taking me to get electric shock, that they have a damp rag they plan on stuffing in my mouth.
I think, It's 2022, how can they just abduct me off the street and make me undergo this torture, and abandon my son in this crowd?
Then I think, it's 2022, so that's exactly what's going to happen.

I bring the letter to the next few sessions, a piece of creased white paper that rests unopened beside the computer, like Mallarmé's ideal poem.

For whatever reason, we never get to it.

I don't know if this non-engagement is part of the therapy, or if she has just forgotten about it.

Eventually she retires as well, so I put the letter away and don't look at it for the next two years.

At an event at a university, C on the panel with me.

I examine my jaw in the bathroom mirror before the event begins, as the pain is so intense I feel certain it must be visible, necrotic.

It's not.

Onstage, C leans over from her wheelchair and whispers, *Are you in pain.*

I nod.

Then, *Are you frightened.*

I nod again, even if I myself would not have thought to use that word.

She nods and takes my hand under the table, a silent tableau we maintain as the auditorium fills with bodies and chatter.

I try to tell people about Plath, about how much she hated the electric shock.

I try to tell the story in a dramatic fashion, using details I've learned from the new biography.
I feel like, if my listener really understood the gravity, Plath's fate might be altered.
I tell E about it at their birthday dinner and I can tell I'm not capturing their attention, probably due to the din of the restaurant, plus some Boston class and sexuality shit that would totally make sense but which I am also probably projecting.
It makes me sad, like I'm failing something larger than myself.
Later that night I dream about the pram in Plath's apartment – white, upright, note attached.

I say that C took my hand, but really her injury had deprived her fingers of their grip, so it's more like, she made a cradle for my hand to rest in – a mini pietà – bringing to mind her adolescent apprenticeship in foot-washing.

At my Buddhist discussion group at the dying sangha, which will die for good during Covid, a male teacher uses as an example during his lecture on attraction the feeling of being excited by a hot girl walking by on the street.

I spend the rest of the class transfixed by my feelings.

In my life as a university professor, I would never say such a thing. But here he's the teacher, and I'm the student.

I don't feel like going up to him after class and saying, That was a fucked-up example, even if I think it was.

It also seems brazen, as the organisation has been racked by sexist scandal, so you'd think the teachers might be shopping around for new material.

That said, I'm sure he did think she was hot, and it was probably a serviceable example of dealing with daily attraction, both for him, and for other people in the room.

Also, I get so tired of people talking about straight men as the only ones walking around with dirty minds.

I rarely find anyone hot in public, but I don't necessarily think this is a virtue.

I think it has more to do with how LA doesn't really have a public, how there is no subway ride wherein you have time to develop feelings about strangers.

And now, of course, no one goes anywhere – my new discussion group is a grid of dimly lit seekers, propped up against our headboards.

The new task, wrought nearly overnight by the virus: surrendering to solitary pain management.

This change is not entirely unwelcome – often I had imagined what it would feel like to just give up, especially as my quest for relief had begun to feel almost recreational, so few were its practical rewards.

Still, giving up on a pain puzzle is not as easy as giving up on certain other things.

Pain pretends urgency; one has to become cold-hearted to its entreaties.

Every day, before logging onto my son's Zoom school –
We can't go on like this / That's what you think.
I am talking to myself, a fractal interiority.
I try to become interested in other interiorities, like that of the dishwasher.
I examine the eggshell caught in the whipping arm, the inscrutable silver disc floating at the machine's navel.
I wonder if, by sheer force of attention, I could render the dishwasher interesting.
Maybe I could write a prose poem, or a series of prose poems, about it, like Ponge.

'The question is not what you look at but how you look & whether you see,' Thoreau wrote in his journal, 1851.

I believe this, but the fact is that magic feels like it is seeping out of my life.

I look for it, I write about it, I read books about it, I talk about it in public (or whatever public Zoom has to offer).

But inside I feel abandoned by it, dispossessed.

I know I am not alone: each morning I read articles about how the pandemic is killing contingency, coincidence, surprise, defamiliarisation – in short, all the conditions that make magic possible.

Yet my failure to summon it feels uniquely my own.

I think about Mother Teresa, who proselytised about the miraculous presence of Christ for decades, when inside she felt bereft – faithless, even.

'Jesus has a very special love for you,' she wrote a friend. '[But] as for me – The silence and the emptiness is so great – that I look and do not see.'

From the grid, I ask a different Buddhist teacher – a female teacher I selected for the no-nonsense vibe I got from her online photo – what she makes of the previous teacher's comment.

She says the sutras are full of suggestions to male monks as to how

to meditate on female corpses, or on women filled with pus, in order to stifle their desire.
She says it's simply disgusting, and I delight in her decree.

The closet detective, the girl who can't stop peeking under the bandage, still fantasises a procedure by which the sensation – which today is shaped like a mean, black bobby pin – could simply be plucked out, as one would excise a rotten limb from Cavity Sam. After all, ten days ago, a team removed a cyst from my left ovary which contained – as we had hoped – nothing but hair, teeth and fat globules, the tangled makings of a changeling.
It is harder to operate on the part of the body responsible for mastication and the generation of speech.
Especially if no scan has revealed a rottenness.

Eventually H tells me that every night I have fallen asleep with our son – which has been nearly every night since he was born – he hears the same soft ping of abandonment that I hear.
Every night he thinks, *Maybe tonight she'll come find me; I guess she's not coming; I guess I'm on my own.*
His late-night party is a dirge.

The first texts tell me that C is in the hospital, admitted for a urinary tract infection that won't clear.
This is not immediately alarming – since her accident, C has had a suprapubic tube susceptible to infections.
This is the tube that I was always so fearful to deal with, terrified, as I was, to send a single fleck of bacteria into her body.
2004, a few months after the accident: J is demonstrating what needs to be done with the tube, telling me how crucial it is to don gloves and sanitise correctly.
I speak from my panic and heart to say, *I'm sorry, but I just don't think I'm cut out for this*.
J looks at me with as much contempt as I've ever seen her muster – maybe not all the way to contempt, but resolve bordering on contempt – and says, *You think any of us were 'cut out for this'? You just do it, that's all*.
Chastened, I did it. And kept doing it.

I call H from our house, where a bunch of people are over at a pool party and I'm tired of hosting them.
A girl with a European purr answers his cell phone, says he can't talk now because of the performance.
He's performing? I ask. Or other people are performing?

Yes, yes, she says, it will disrupt the performance.
Look, I say, this is his wife and I need to talk to him right now.
Oh, perfect, she says, it's over now, here he is.
He comes in tender.
I say I've had it with his being away, I miss him, this is ridiculous, can he please come home.
Yes, yes, he says, he'll be home in twenty minutes.
I realise then that he will probably be bringing home Covid, how could he not.
I think to myself, I never feel well, I am never well.
Something is systemically wrong with me, maybe I'm systemically sick.
Even in my sleep I tell myself, That's not true, it's just a fear, it's your anxiety talking, you do sometimes feel well, maybe even often.
Our dog comes over to comfort me but instead of being a nine-pound white poodle she's a medium-sized dog made of nubby green fabric, a replicant.

Watching the waiter refill my sparkling water from a cobalt bottle, I'm moved to tears – it seems so decadent, so kind.
It's the first time I've been away from home alone in over two years, and while I know my happiness risks making me come across as

overeager, it feels too good to care – so I break one of my cardinal rules, and tell my lunchmate, a smart writer whom I've heretofore met only on Zoom, about an unrealised writing idea.

He laughs, *So you're telling me your next book is going to be about your dishwasher?*

It had sounded potentially interesting in the privacy of my mind; in his mouth, in this mirthful eatery, it sounds like the story of a mom with a sponge, *a fun sponge.*

As I cycle through my shame – visible, as always, on my face – I realise that the magic isn't in the dishwasher – it's in the bloodjet, the mortifying abundance of telling.

It's just like Freud's theory of dreams – it's not the dream that matters, it's the telling of the dream – the words you choose, the risks you take in externalising your mind.

This is Freud's 'talking cure' – Freud, who died of jaw cancer, for which he had over thirty debilitating and disfiguring oral surgeries.

The next text drops into the pit: a scan has revealed tumours on C's pancreas, and elsewhere.

Everyone knows what that means.

J tells me that C was very clear with the doctor: I'm not afraid to die, but I don't want any more pain.

I am impressed by her bravery, and sorrowful at everything that has driven her to this statement.

Seventeen years of pain, more than enough and more than too much then more than enough and too much again.

I talk to J on the phone, she is imagining there might be time for people to say goodbye, and because she is an excellent planner she is already planning how to do it in the midst of Covid, in a freezing Connecticut winter.

The vaccines are not out yet, the winter is caked in grimness and fear and death.

She imagines setting C up in her wheelchair in their backyard, even if it's freezing out – no problem, she'll rent heat lamps – and receiving tearful visitors.

As J is speaking I know that none of this is going to happen.

I don't know if I know this because I actually know it or because I fear it; I've learned that a lot of things I think I know are just things I fear.

But I also know that whatever I know or don't know, J needs to imagine this scene.

So I say That sounds right, I will help plan it, I will be there.

That night I can barely sleep – there is a storm that howls, periodically irradiating the grey-orange sky with lightning – so I hear the sirens right away.

It's a fire across the street, at the Spanish where an older couple lives with their daughter, a disabled woman in her fifties.
By dawn the whole block is cordoned off by fire trucks and ambulances, the rainy morning streaked with red and blue lights.
I watch from my porch wrapped up in a blanket while my son sleeps.
The parents are standing in their front yard with raincoats draped around their shoulders when their daughter is carried out on a stretcher covered by black tarps.
I don't want to leave my son to go comfort them and I doubt they want me, a stranger, to do so, but it feels terrible to watch them standing alone in the rain, firefighters wandering around their charred property, their daughter's body being loaded into an ambulance with their house still steaming.
Maybe it feels extra terrible because I once watched my father get carried away from the Blithedale house under the same tarps, a moment I have come to regard as the navel of all loneliness.
I contemplate this dismal tableau until my son wakes up, then rummage around for cheer, drop the needle onto the Windham Hill acoustic guitar LP from my childhood that has become our home-school soundtrack, and prepare the day's whiteboard.
I decorate his schedule with the same aesthetic gimmicks I employed when I was a waitress charged with rendering the evening's menu into chalk.
It was sort of a contest between us — which waitress could make the nicest-looking board, to get the customers to buy up.

I go see a dentist with a lovely office – potted plants, rows of clean chairs, state-of-the-art equipment.
She says she doesn't need to X-ray my mouth as she can already tell what's wrong.
She hands me a mouthpiece made of fat black rubber which fits over the top of my front teeth like a boxer's guard.
I put it in and despite its ugliness – it looks like I'm sporting a tyre, my upper lip unnaturally puffed out – it's perfect, all the pain evaporates right away.
I walk a couple of times around an outdoor track to test it out, then thank her and go on my way.

C's moment of clarity with the doctor proves fleeting: her sodium is high and her ammonia is low and she's losing lucidity, plus the pain meds – she never speaks again.
She is actively dying – this after being admitted to the hospital a few days ago with a cancer no one knew she had.
J tells me that the doctors utter the sentence, *The cancer is progressing by the hour.*
I didn't even know that was a thing.
I feel boxed in: I want to get on a plane to be by her, to be there for these final hours, just as I flew to her right after her accident.
In fact it feels like I have to – to bookend the pain, this friendship,

this love, which has meant everything to me and somehow lies at the core of who I am.

But I know that even if I could get there they wouldn't let me into the hospital – even J had to get a 'compassionate exception' – and I can't take my son with me or leave him behind, so I'm stuck in my living room with these incoming texts reporting C's stunningly swift decline.

Only J is there to bear witness and shoulder it, as it has so often been.

I'm reading my phone in the morning dark when I hear a noise outside.

I look out onto the driveway and see a hooded figure in the driver's seat of my car.

For a minute I think it's H, then I realise it's not.

The driveway runs alongside the house, so he's about ten feet from me, fucking with the wires.

I duck down, scared that he might have seen me.

I don't want to lose my car, and I'm afraid to be here with my son with this stranger so nearby, so I call the police.

I stay low for another hour. No police come.

Now it's light out and the man has gone.

The car is pillaged but still there; it's New Year's Day.
My son tumbles out of bed and I am so happy, as always, to see him.

Please send me pictures of what's happening, I text, and so J does.
In the first, C is lying on her side, her grey hair very thin, black onyx studs in her ears, as if she had been at the opera and somehow found herself here instead, in a hospital bed with a heart-shaped, orange-and-purple fleece pillow beside her head, a white washcloth folded under her mouth.

A few hours later, two squad cars pull up, and three cops theatrically pull out their guns to 'secure the property'.
They scoff at me when I say I may have left the car unlocked.
The whole thing feels like a farce; I hate them and I hate myself for calling them.

I go down the Google hole, and discover that Susan Olsen (Cindy) has gone full MAGA, was fired in 2016 from a podcast for sending a gay actor a message that read, 'Hey there little pussy, let me get my big boy pants on and Reallly take you on!!! What a snake in the grass you are you lying piece of shit too cowardly to confront me in real life so you do it on Facebook. You are the biggest faggot ass in the world the biggest pussyy! My Dick is bigger than yours Which ain't sayin much! What a true piece of shit you are! Lying faggot! I hope you meet your karma SLOWLY AND PAINFULLY.'

I keep this update to myself, its little snow globe of sorrow.

The next night, the burnt-up house gets ransacked.
I guess some folks scour the news feeds for fires, just to make sure other folks lose everything.

J calls early in the morning and says it's time to say goodbye.
Says she's going to put the phone up to C's ear, and I should say what I have to say.
I'm not cut out for this kind of thing, I want to say, but we've been through that before.
C's breathing is loud and laboured; all of her personhood is audible in the rattle.

I remember that she told the doctor just days ago that she wasn't afraid to die, but that she didn't want any more pain, so I tell her this is the hard part, that she's about to get free.

I think of her flying off her bicycle on the day of her accident, flying through the air in the woods, and how that day she landed, whereas this time she's not going to land.

This time, her undoing will be final.

I love you so much, you are surrounded by love, this is the hard part, you're about to fly free.

I keep talking but feel weirdly insecure, like, should I say different things or just keep repeating the same things, when will J take the phone back, does it matter any more that C knows how much she is loved, or will too much love act as a tether impeding her departure.

I am wondering these things as I keep talking and listening to C's rattle, then J takes the phone back and it's over.

She has more calls to make; my turn is done.

I'm texting with J while sitting on the couch with my son watching *The Great Pottery Throw Down*.

It's raku week; we love raku.

We love how the head judge weeps every time he feels moved by a contestant's ceramic achievement – each time he tears up, we tear up, too.

J sends a photo in which I can see the change – C's eyes have crusted over, her skin is waxen and bluish, she is going.
I feel sick and out of time, yet I am trying to be in my body with my son on the couch talking about the challenges of tossing horsehair onto vases in an ash pit.
I catalogue sensations as I've been taught: his soft skin next to me, the sweet cotton of his pyjamas, the softness of the plush blanket, my feet rubbing against the inside of my socks.
I worry that if I cry at the beauty of the raku I will never stop.

In the middle of the following night, another photo arrives: *She's gone*.
Eyes half open, deranged and empty eye sockets, cobalt rock where there had once been sky blue.
The orange-and-purple fleece heart pillow pokes out of the sheet next to her head like an anime companion.
She's gone.

I sponge off the whiteboard and write with a fat, grape-scented marker:
January 6, 2021 !!
8.30–9 a.m.: Morning Meeting !!

9–10 a.m.: Read Aloud !!
10–12 p.m.: Home Stewardship !!
12–1 p.m.: Lunch !!
1–2 p.m.: Choice !!
2–2.30 p.m.: Farewell !!

J sends me a photo of C taken on Christmas Day, of C about to delve into a festive bowl of sweet potato soup with her ergonomic spoon.
This was twelve days ago, J writes. *What happened?*
What happened, indeed.
I border the day's rectangle with flowers and vines, keep the TV on all day at low volume, the remote close at hand, in case of live butchery at the Capitol.

A few days after C dies, H comes home to visit.
We don't embrace, out of respect for our 'pods' – we sit on the porch in chairs set the requisite distance apart while I weep convulsively.
I know he is taking these spells away to take care of someone else, but today that knowledge has fled the sieve – I blame him for C's death, for the distance between us, for the convulsive weeping with no one to hold me.

I can't stop hearing C's voice saying, 'Maggie, my dear Maggie.'
No one will ever say my name like that again – no lover, no parent, no husband, no friend.
The way C knew me died with her; from now on I will be less loved, less known.

The best part of 'remote schooling' is when we turn it off.
Sometimes, to my son's glee, I snap the computer shut before the lesson is over, as when an instructor was valiantly trying to walk us through a complex Chrome download while wearing the filter of a corgi.
Liberated, we head to the arroyo, where we amass piles of fallen pepper berries, take pictures of scat, and spin helicopter seeds through the chain-link fence, launching them down to the trickle of LA river below.

At a party at E's house, though it wasn't really E's house, which will always be East 3rd Street, but a place they were renting in Koreatown.
There were a lot of hip people there I didn't know so it felt intimidating and alien, the way most things in LA felt to me back then.

It was so painful to have moved from New York City, where I'd
spent my entire adult life, to this place where I couldn't read the
environment, didn't know the characters in the play.
People would say, Do you want to go see some art?
And next thing you knew you were in some corn maze that an artist
collective had planted between a Metro facility and Chinatown,
multiple freeways away from 'home'.
Beyond the fact that I'd hit a spiritual bottom, I also had to quit
drinking just so that I could find my way home each night without
crashing my car, which would have been scary and humiliating, not to
mention proof that I was the alcoholic I'd always feared myself to be.

We hadn't come to the party together but we planned on leaving
together.
I was going to follow your filthy, pale-blue, biodiesel Mercedes
(later totalled in LAX's Lot C) to the basement in which you were
squatting, the basement of Uncle Silas's house on El Paso.
From across the room you sent a text to my flip phone saying you
had picked up some lube – texts were so new then we didn't even
say text, we said 'word', as in, 'I sent you a word message'.
I knew then that you wanted me as much as I wanted you, a chaotic
and explosive feeling that fuels the birth of worlds.

I am supposed to give a reading at the New York Public Library – it's something big, all the Supreme Court justices are going to be there.

I am confused about whether we're supposed to wear masks.

The chair of my department is telling me animatedly – hysterically almost – that the youth have been requesting that I read poems from *Jane*, in particular the one about how I tried to arm myself against imaginary predators with a butcher knife.

I think, if Amy Coney Barrett is going to be there, I have to read the poem about how *we've fooled ourselves, / we who've split blood into that which pollutes, and that which redeems.*

I feel deeply angry – Roe angry.

Suddenly I feel a huge weird pop in my mouth.

I go to the bathroom and see that my tongue is bloody in the centre and I've lost a front tooth.

This is disturbing, but it at least explains the pain.

It doesn't explain what happens next, however, which is that a lower front tooth that's been sticking up a bit suddenly pops up and out – more blood.

The remaining teeth shift and fill the spot, it doesn't look that weird.

But then it happens again, and again.

It occurs to me that I'm going to lose all my bottom teeth this way, that they're on a conveyor belt to their destruction.

Each one leaves behind sharp stringy black hairs, like fur.

And yet – as soon as we left the party and pulled onto Olympic Boulevard, you started driving too quickly for me to follow, pulling through yellow lights, changing lanes without warning.

Why would you be trying to lose me, or why would you not care about losing me, right when you were trying – or so I thought! – to find me?

It was one of those moments you come back to again and again, turning it over like the Arkenstone, like – if only you could have known how confused and forsaken I felt out there on the boulevard, maybe we could have kept such moments from recurring, stacking up. Or, if only I had known more of what you were thinking – were you trying to impress me? Did you think I knew the way? Or was it just too hard to keep everything in mind?

If we could – if I could – finally understand, maybe this terrible and terribly familiar feeling would finally lift, of someone who says they love you and really does seem to desire you but who is running up the road, there's just this one thing I've got to do, this is just who I am, another creature to assist, pinned pupils, attention deficit disorder, another lover, arteriosclerosis, progressing by the hour, up and over the horizon line, gone.

I examine the hairs, and realise there is a fur tumour under my chin that is pushing up on my teeth, that's the real problem, and if I survive I will be radically disfigured.

I think about Roger Ebert, and the challenge of being known
for sharing your opinions in public, then having to undergo the
dispossession of your jaw, your chin, your throat, your capacity to
speak.
In the meantime, I still have to get to the reading, but I haven't eaten.
I ask someone to order me a hamburger, which I eat messily while
going through piles and piles of old poems.
I want to find something that will humiliate ACB, even though I
know that, even if I do, it won't undo what's been done.
None of the poems is finished – they're just marked-up drafts, all the
edits yet to be entered.

*I'm afraid I'm going to be married but sleep alone for the rest of
my life* – a sentence I disinter from beneath my mouth, from the
undermaw.
Its banality is as astounding as its depth.
*It's you I want and have always wanted, please come find me,
neither of us has to be this alone.*

On a road trip with Alice.
We're in the south, Missouri, it's afternoon, and we see fat hairy
spinning tornados near where a hot-air balloon event is beginning.

People in the hot-air balloons are competing with the tornados – it's dangerous.
Later we hear a woman has died.
We take shelter in a dark wood Airbnb, where I get the attic, the one Greg moves into when he gets groovy.
Alice calls from the lower house, says she is super disappointed in me, that I made Cindy far more scared about the tornados than she needed to be.
She's just a kid, she says.
She starts going on and on and really laying into me and I feel annoyed because Alice is not a mother and so I say, Look, I'm going to stop you right there.
I register that you think I upset Cindy, and I'm sorry for that. Mothers aren't perfect in their efforts to look out for all potential harms and also not freak themselves or their children out, and clearly I failed in your eyes here.
I'll likely fail a bunch more times and then cross my fingers that when he sets out I did enough right; God knows I love him more than I've ever loved anyone or anything, and at some point you have to trust that all that love will outweigh or at least balance out all your defects and mistakes, as love is what makes us safe above and beyond safety.
Alice gets teary and asks if I'm going to remove her from the show, which I apparently control.
I tell her that I've seen her be strong and demanding with male showrunners and agents, that she's way ahead of her time.

I tell her that I'm just a Marcia (suddenly I *am* Marcia), slight and blonde, and that all the parts I'll be able to get will be beneath me. As I speak I know what's to come – the Quaaludes, the selling of sex for drugs – it's unclear if Alice knows, too.

April 13, 2020

Dear Maggie,

How's it going kiddo? I've missed you so much. It's so good to talk to you, it's been so long. I'm so proud of you. I wish I could give you a huge hug. You've really gotten 'more substantial'!

A few things. First, I never wanted to leave you and your sister. I don't know what happened to me – it was swift and then I was gone. If I could have chosen, I would have stayed with you for as long as you lived. I would be seventy-six today – we could have had so much more time. I wish we had had that time. I didn't abandon you – I loved you girls so much, I loved life so much, I would never have chosen to go. It was not something I could control. Please don't ever forget that.

Second, I have always been with you. At every big moment, and even the small ones, I am with you. I am so proud of you. I know your talents and, more than that, I know your heart. Your humour. Your essential goodness. We are part of each other, and nothing will ever change that. If you've ever felt scared or alone, or whenever you do, remember at that very moment that I didn't leave you, that I'm with you, that I am a part of you, and that we are love.

Third, dying isn't the worst thing in the world. It really is part of the cycle of life, and it makes life precious. Don't be frightened of what lies ahead for us all. I've passed through this world, and it's okay. You don't need to be afraid of doing the same.

Fourth, you will be all right. You have been all right. You are all right. It was so hard for you, when I died, and there have been some hard moments since. You're in one right now, I see. You have all the fortitude you need to get through it. Some of that fortitude is yours alone, but some of it is the Nelson spirit – a certain *joie de vivre* coupled with hard work and passionate energy. It's 'the force', as we used to say, and you have it. Don't give up on the world or yourself or anyone in it. Life is beautiful and painful and precious – I miss it, and I miss you. Enjoy it in whatever its form.

I have to go now, but remember how much time I spent laughing and smiling, dancing and loving, playing the guitar and singing, teasing you and cuddling you. Love your son just as well, and don't worry so much about trying to control fate. You don't always have to try so hard. You are doing your absolute best, I see and salute it.

Remember the song we used to sing, try not to try too hard, it's just a lovely ride. It's really true.

Love always,

Your dad.

I go back to the last dentist I saw before Covid.
I return to him because I remember having liked him, and having been somewhat impressed that his no-frills approach of naproxen, compresses, stretches and soft-food diet was as effective as it was. Also, he didn't shame me about my various adventures, even as he told me that he had spent the better part of a decade trying to get the board to ban practices such as those used by the dentist in the valley.

He re-examines my mouth, and says its measurements are unchanged from my visit three years ago.
I have difficulty reconciling this observation with my sense that my mouth has been rearranging itself daily, catastrophically.
He says I have an exceptionally strong bite force, and that it's not unusual for people with my particular dental arrangement to have jaw pain.

I leave his office feeling buoyant, and in no rush to restart his programme.

I'm still in pain, but I want to pause over the fact that, rather than feeling gaslit by the gap between my internal experience and my body's outward stats, I feel momentarily calmed by it.

When I was in labour with my son, my birth coach kept encouraging me to notice the space between contractions – she said I needed to notice the space so that I could use it as a reprieve, to gear up for the next contraction, to stay strong.

I remember thinking, there is a life lesson here, but this isn't the moment for it.

Around the second anniversary of C's death, J tells me she's been noticing a shift in her grief, from inestimable sorrow at all she has lost, to the recognition that it is within her power to offer the world at least some of what C offered us – the presence, the rigour, the holding.

As J says this I realise that a similar feeling has been growing inside me as well, no words, just a little bulge of light nudging out.

For the first time in over two decades of being a teacher, I recognise that I am one.

I really tried, but the truth is that I couldn't feel the pauses between contractions – maybe because I was too disoriented by the pain each one left in its wake, and too fearful of the one I knew was coming. The moment for the lesson is now.

Thank you

Joshua Beckman & Wave Books, once and again

Michal Shavit & Fern Press

Brian Blanchfield ~ Miranda July ~ Ben Lerner ~ PJ Mark ~
Anthony McCann: the like-tongued

& the magical creatures with whom I shared heart and home during this time.

Disclaimer

This work conjoins dream and reality; all representations of people, places and events should be understood in that spirit.